JUICING RECIPES FOR VITALITY AND HEALTH

BY: DREW CANOLE

FitLife.TV

Publishing services provided by **Archangel Ink**

ISBN: 1517272890
ISBN-13: 978-1517272890

Drew Canole, Star of FitLife.TV

Visit www.FitLife.TV/kindlevideo in your web browser for a personal (and funny) message from Drew right now.

Hi, my friend. Drew Canole here. If you picked up this book, I am guessing you have a passion for health and more specifically, a passion for juicing—something that has changed my life and that of thousands of others.

When I started juicing, the idea of drinking fruits and vegetables seemed strange. But after having my first glass and instantly feeling the positive effects of my cells coming to life, I knew I had to go down the rabbit hole and understand what was happening inside of my body and how I could share it with as many people as possible.

I know the world of health can be confusing. Trust me, I've been where you may be now. With so much information available to us nowadays, what are we supposed to believe?

My goal is to take the confusion out of juicing and help you better understand WHY you should juice and how exactly it affects your body, including your physical and emotional state, even your mental clarity, skin, and hormones! Juicing is powerful, my friend and I am proof that making small changes over time can pay off . . . big time!

Are you ready to transform?

Remember, we're in this together.

Drew

Join the juicing movement at <u>Facebook.com/vegetablejuicing</u>

Table of Contents

A Juice-Fueled Journey

My sincere hope is that this book changes your life. No matter what your overall health goal is, or where you are in your journey, juicing has the potential to reshape not only your physical landscape, but also your internal workings as well. Ever hear of the expression, "Green on the inside, clean on the inside?" Well, my friend . . . it's true!

Simply drinking even one fresh-pressed green juice each day has the power to supply your body with the essential vitamins, nutrients, and minerals it needs for sustained energy, vitality, and overall health.

Some major benefits of juicing are that:

- they are super easy to make and take just minutes to prepare (ingredients can even be prepped beforehand and stored to grab and use in a hurry);
- they are made in your own kitchen, so you know exactly what's in them;
- they supply your body with massive amounts of nutrients that you need to feel your best from the inside out;
- you will feel the power of raw energy once the juice hits your bloodstream, leaving you feeling energized all day long;
- the right combinations help to decrease inflammation and combat disease.

One of the foremost reasons I was able to go from 17 percent body fat down to sub-7 percent was because of juicing. Not *that* kind of juicing—I'm talking straight-up, 100 percent pure "green" veggie juice. And maybe an occasional apple or other fruit to sweeten things up a bit.

I was first turned on to juicing by my good friend, William Ripley. He told me the devastating tale of his heroic father who had recently suffered a heart attack. The doctors had given him a very short time to live—*unless* he were to make some pretty radical changes immediately. At the time, his father was severely overweight, his testosterone (a critical hormone) was at an all-time low, and he had very little, if any, energy whatsoever. What's sad is that 70 percent of the population suffers in the same way as Mr. Ripley. The good news is that YOU DON'T HAVE TO!

Determined to get better, Mr. Ripley set out to find a solution to his failing health. He visited multiple doctors and tried various homeopathic remedies, along with an expansive array of other methods for healing. He was at a friend's house when he shared his bad news and explained his situation to her. Determined and desperate, he asked her for advice. All that he could think about was the prognosis—*death*—and the fact that he wasn't ready to go without a fight.

In that very moment, she pulled out a juicer from her small pantry and gathered veggies from her fridge. As she washed the vegetables, Mr. Ripley started to chuckle.

"What are we going to do with *those*?" he asked.

Mr. Ripley's friend's response was simple. "We are going to juice them!"

Mr. Ripley was unfamiliar with the concept of juicing vegetables, but because he was desperate and ready to do whatever it would take to be well, he agreed to give it a try. Simply put: he was running out of time. Every heartbeat was another gift from God. Each thump reminded him of the years of self-sabotage and abuse he'd subjected himself to, including years of poor sleeping habits and a highly toxic diet. Thankfully, Mr. Ripley was open for a change that day.

The juice his friend made for him consisted of a couple of carrots, a cucumber, and some ginger. She handed the cup to him and he grimaced. He had always had a disdain for the taste of carrots and had never even tasted raw ginger. But he put the glass up to his lips and took his first sip.

"This stuff tastes amazing!" he proclaimed.

She smiled and reflected on how often she had seen this expression from newbie juicers.

After Mr. Ripley's first juice, and with the hope of losing weight and regaining his health, he became a juicing addict. Not only did he start juicing three times a day, he convinced all of his neighbors to juice. They were hesitant to take him up on his invitations at first, but they decided to give it a try out of respect and support, since they wanted to keep their friend around as long as possible.

Months went by and Mr. Ripley—remaining faithful to his new love of juicing—felt more energy coursing through his veins and began to drop the excess weight—*and quickly!*—like he had the metabolism of a prepubescent adolescent.

Eventually, the medication prescribed by his cardiologist started giving him problems. He explained to his doctor that it was causing him to vomit and convulse. The doctor quickly responded by running tests. A few hours later, the doctor came back in with his results. It seemed that Mr. Ripley's immune system had strengthened so much that it had formed a "block" against the medicine.

His doctor wanted to increase the dosage of the medicine, but Mr. Ripley knew that he no longer needed it and knew that it wasn't the medicine that was improving his health and keeping him alive. It was the juice!

He had to get the secret out!

And fortunately, he did.

Transformation Story

"Since doing Alpha Reset, I am down 25 pounds! I have a ton more energy and have fallen in love with moving my body again. I sleep better, my skin is clear, I have more focus and wake up every morning excited to start the day. This program has been one of the greatest gifts that I have ever given myself and I am soooooo happy to have been able to share it with you all. The stats are fantastic, but THE GREATEST joy for me is that I have met all of the transformation goals that I wrote down on the application for this program . . . "

—Angela B.

Inspiration Strikes

After his eldest son, William, shared his father's heart wrenching story with me, I realized that I had to get a juicer—ASAP! While I wasn't in as poor shape as Mr. Ripley (yet), I knew that the way I had been treating my body over the years was only setting me up to be another sad statistic and I knew that I wanted to live a better life. This decision would end up being the best investment for my health that I'd ever make.

At the time, I had lots of energy but was constantly searching for the nearest coffee shop for my caffeine fix. I was in good physical shape but nowhere near where I wanted to be. I would often work out twice a day, sometimes for more than three hours a day. Regardless, I just couldn't lose what looked like baby fat surrounding my abdominal region and my little chipmunk face.

Maybe you can relate to this.

Like many people, I was severely dehydrated and didn't even know it. Often I would mistake my dehydration for hunger, which forced me to overeat, choosing the wrong foods for my body and leaving me feeling sluggish and unmotivated. For years this went on and instead of drinking nourishing liquids, I would overeat pizza and other life-draining foods. This is the story of most of the population. We are "the dehydrated nation" and also the most overweight. Do you think there is a connection?

Well I am here to tell you . . . there is—a big one, in fact!

As a culture, we load up on soda, coffee, sugar-laden tea, alcohol, and other beverages that are not good for our physical well-being. One twenty-ounce bottle of Coke has the equivalent of sixteen packets of sugar in it, yet we wonder why America is fighting an obesity/diabetes epidemic, which is a leading cause of death in America.

FACT: There is a recommended limit for sugar consumption and in the United States, it's estimated that we are consuming *3– 5 times* that amount. A simple reminder to track of this is: 1 tsp is equal to 4 grams of sugar. Women should not consume more than 6 tsp (24 grams) daily and men should not consume more than 9 tsp (36 grams) daily[1]. And unfortunately, sugar is hidden in just about everything.

But that's for another day. Just be aware of the fact that this poison you're ingesting daily is causing ailments that are in fact avoidable, such as acne, fatigue, digestion issues, mood disorders, chronic inflammation . . . even disease!

---

[1]
http://www.heart.org/HEARTORG/GettingHealthy/NutritionCenter/HealthyEating/Sugar-101_UCM_306024_Article.jsp

It's no coincidence that the most common diseases in the US are diet-related, some of which include diabetes (type 2), cancer, heart disease and obesity. We are eating out of convenience and making unwise decisions when it comes to our long-term health. It takes the body more energy to process this fat-laden, sugar-loaded, processed, lifeless junk and we are giving ourselves less time to heal.

Through a rigorous juicing schedule, within three months, I started to see a six-pack peeking through my abs that I had never seen on myself before. This was enough to encourage the beginning of a lifelong habit, using food to transform my body and, ultimately, my entire life!

Some of the transforming results that juicing brought to my life—and to that of many others I've since spoken with—were:

- More energy
- More chiseled muscle
- Healthier hormone levels
- Healthier skin and hair
- More apparent overall glow
- Greater mental acuteness
- Sexiness (juicing is super sexy!)
- *A MUCH HAPPIER (and healthier) DREW!*

Would you like to have any of these things in your life? If you answered "yes," then it is time to learn about one of the greatest discoveries I've made up until this point.

Let me help you "Juice Up Your Life!"

Transformation Story

"I lost 10 pounds, 3 inches off my hips and 3.5 inches off my waist. I am way less bloated, feel very energized and am working towards a better exercise routine. I loved all the attention we received and the support from Mae and Jill and the inspiration from the group members."

—Linda F.

Interested in group coaching?

Go here for details: http://bit.ly/1hHx64t

Why Should You Juice?

"All the smart and healthy kids are doing it."

A nd by "kids," I mean when you juice, you feel younger, more energized, and ALIVE—like a kid again. But don't take my word for it! You have to experience it for yourself; no one can fully capture what juicing can do for you until you have savored your first cup and felt the undeniable effects and the amazing power of GREENS, extracted at their cellular level to provide you an immense amount of vitamins, minerals, and nutrients that your body so desperately craves.

Since you probably don't have a glass of fresh vegetable juice in front of you now, let me explain the multitude of health benefits, regardless of your age, race, or current physical condition.

It has been said that we are what we eat and it has been proven that a diet of fresh juice (not store-bought), legumes, healthy fats, quality protein, and organic fruits and vegetables will aid you in obtaining great health. I consider myself living proof!

This book is not to be treated as a scientific research paper based on the thousands of trials and tests done on humans for decades on end. No, this book is about my own personal experience with juicing and the many others who have joined *The New Lean* revolution in order to take ownership once and for all of their physical and mental well-being. Health is about embracing and challenging all aspects of the mind, body, and spirit. Juicing is a great starting point to cultivate a brighter future in all of these vitally important areas.

I believe that by adding fresh vegetable juice to your life, you will contribute greatly to your cardiovascular health, among other things. As I sit here typing this, my resting heart rate is anywhere from forty-five to fifty beats a minute. If you apply the principles in this book to your own life, you will enhance your physical performance, help your blood pressure, gain restful sleep, and increase your energy—more than you could have possibly ever imagined!

I've had many friends join me on various social media networks, asking for juice recipes and then going out and buying juicers. I receive a steady flow of e-mails from people who have joined the revolution and who have freed themselves from destructive habits and failing health.

Every day, my friends and I are nourishing trillions of cells in our bodies with the best form of food we could ever take in. I'm not advocating that you stop eating food and drink only juice. What I am suggesting, however, is to plan out five to eight small meals a day and enjoy fresh green juice in between. My small meals are basically snacks. This keeps my insulin from spiking and my metabolism revved up to the max. When your metabolism is working *for* you and not *against* you, you can stop worrying about working out so much and counting calories and focus on supporting your body with whole food nutrition and mindful movement.

My body was laden with pounds of excess fat and I thought the only way to rid myself of this was to work out—*a lot*. Boy, was I wrong. Now, I work out half as much and my body takes care of itself. Once all the toxins were removed from my system, it was much easier to lose the fat in those seemingly impossible-to-lose places. I feel lighter, more vibrant, and limitless. You can too!

I finally transformed—and I did it the right way! No diets or starvation, just good old fashioned FOOD, while keeping my body active and fueled for energy and success.

Transformation Story

"Here are my results from the 30 Day Detox - I lost: 17 pounds, lots of inches, fat stores as confirmed by my MD via ketone measurement, 25 points off my total cholesterol, 8 points off my triglycerides, 29 points off my LDL 'bad' cholesterol, 20 points off my fasting blood sugar, sugar cravings and otherwise feeling controlled by food, bloating and frequent stomach aches. What I gained: 7 points on my HDL 'good' cholesterol, the healthiest pulses I've had in 3 years of acupuncture treatments, the skills to make a variety of whole, healthy meals without any processed foods or added sugar, tons of new nutritional knowledge, a sharpened ability to tune into what my body needs, great sleep and the ability to wake up early and get out of bed with ease before the alarm, increased physical strength, softer, clear, brighter skin, old clothes that fit again, increased confidence in multiple areas, the ability to eat to live instead of living to eat, many new awesome friends! Thank you Mae and Jill and the other ladies for your support and encouragement and of course, you too, Drew!"

—Beth H.

The Benefits of Live Juice

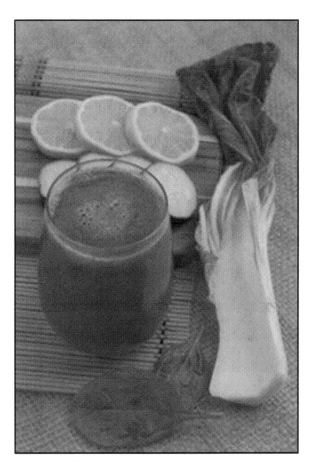

As we all know, we are what we eat. The body needs live food to build live cells. When I say "live foods," I'm talking about foods that come directly out of the soil and are still alive. Raw foods—not cooked or processed—such as beans, nuts, legumes, fruits, and my favorite . . . VEGETABLES (especially the green ones)!

When we eat live foods, our bodies consume the liquid immediately and the pass all of the excess on to the lower digestive tract. Imagine an IV of super-powerful, energy-rich foods pumped immediately into the organ of your choice, supplying all the quintessential nutrients you need for the day. The juicer does all of the work for you, so that when you drink that glass of fresh "heaven in your mouth" (that's what I call it), you feel it instantly! Your cells rejoice!

The juice from the juicer is much better for you than any juice you can buy from the store, or even at the local farmer's market. When juice sits on a counter or in the fridge, it oxidizes and loses the lion's share of nutrients. Plus, juice from a juicer is not pasteurized, meaning it isn't cooked or boiled to help it stay on the shelf longer. The fresh juice is literally bursting with live energy ready to heal, pump, and energize you all day.

Many of my friends first asked me, "Why a juicer? Can't I do the same thing with a blender?" The answer, simply, is "no." Using a blender puts pulp into your juice, which is the same thing as eating the whole thing. And while this pulp—or fiber—is important, your body still has to expend energy to break it down. So while your body does need fiber—and I do advocate eating plenty of fresh fruits and vegetables—the juicer provides you with a cup of pure, unadulterated vitamins and minerals taken from the deepest part of the food you're juicing, allowing your body to soak in all the goodies without the pressure of digestion. Let's face it, sometimes we could all use a break. Your body is no different.

FACT: One cup of raw carrot juice contains the same amount of nutrients as four cups of diced carrots. Carrot juice tastes like a sweet dessert—without the guilt—and leaves you with energy instead of crashing from a sugar rush.

Ninety-five percent of the nourishment from fruit and vegetable juice is immediately released into the bloodstream because there is nothing interfering with the processing once it hits your stomach. Before I started juicing, I would consume enough vitamins and supplements to open a pharmacy. After juicing for a while, I could tell that the vitamins would have to go because I was already supplying my body with all it needed through the juice alone! So, when you consider the costly vitamins that also take up valuable space in your cabinets, it's a no-brainer: move the veggies in and kick out the excess supplements.

Transformation Story

> *"I am down 9 pounds; 1 inch off waist, hips, bust - feeling stronger, more energized, hopeful and optimistic."*
>
> —Robin O.

Veggie vs. Fruit Juice

It's important to know the difference between the two.
Vegetables are much more difficult to digest, but they are also loaded with an immense amount of nutrition. (Don't let this sway you away from them—your body is smart, it knows how to break them down). They tend to be much bulkier and break down slower in the body. When I drink green veggie juice, my mind and body reward me immediately with lasting energy and immunity.

You see, vegetables are the building blocks of life! They are responsible for providing you with strong healthy bones, tissues, muscles, and nerve support. When you consume vegetables, you can rest assured that you are getting all—or most—of the nutrients, minerals and vitamins you need for that day.

Whole fruits are much easier to digest than vegetables and should always be taken separately. If I'm going to indulge in a fruit juice, I'll leave a window of thirty minutes to an hour before I eat or drink anything else. Most fruits—like apples, pears, and plums—contain a lot of digestive enzymes that will keep your digestive system regular. Fruits have the lion's share of the antioxidants your body requires as well, so they are important too.

Fruits give me radical amounts of energy before I make my way into the gym at 6:00 every morning. On occasion, I'll have a cheat day where I skip the gym and eat more carbs than usual, usually rice or potatoes. On these days, I'll prepare my body by drinking fresh grapefruit juice. This helps control my insulin levels, keeping me a lean machine—even on cheat days.

Vegetable juicing is always best when you're trying to lose weight. The minerals and high potassium content hydrate your cells and force out the sodium that causes water retention. Regularly drinking vegetable juice helps super-boost your health and remove toxins in your body.

Many of the green drinks are effective at pushing out excess water and toxins that could be causing your cells to retain fat. For example, the Mega Man Green Drink (included in this book) will get rid of the excess water from your cells. The Mega Man consists of kale, spinach, celery, lemon, dandelion greens, cucumber, and ginger; it's also one of my favorites. This combination is a potassium powerhouse. For taste, you might add half a carrot and a green apple, or maybe a quarter of a lemon. If you don't do anything else to lose weight, at least drink one glass (eight to ten ounces) of this juice every day and see—*and feel*—the difference!

Overall Health Benefits

Eating enough fruits and vegetables can sometimes be difficult given the current demanding workloads and fast-paced lifestyles that we all live. Many of the people who have sat down with me ask me how I have enough time to meditate, juice, eat healthy, run a business, and work out. It's like I'm some kind of freak they found at a circus show. My response to them is simple.

A healthy lifestyle is the foundation for everything! The time I take to better my physical and mental health is the time that gives me my life force for living an amazing life! The time I dedicate to my personal well-being gives me the unstoppable amount of energy I have on a daily basis. It calms me and balances me, and the best part about it is that it keeps me super healthy. Without a healthy mind and body, we are unable to do all that is possible in this life. I get so much more accomplished in my day with this healthy foundation and you will too—you just need to decide and commit to investing in yourself and start doing it!

Transformation Story

"I had an excellent yearly doctor's appointment . . . Weight down 90 pounds, BP perfect and I had an EKG. I got the best compliment from the doc that my heart is as smooth as an athlete! Feeling proud and happy!"

—Doreen C.

Nutrition Benefits of Veggies and Fruit

I wanted to include the nutritional benefits of the ingredients used in the juices I am about to share with you. You see, my friend, real, whole foods are POWERFUL (fruits and veggies, in particular)! Food can either be the best medicine or the worst poison. The good news is that you get to decide how you fuel your incredibly intelligent body!

I encourage you to try new things. Each week, commit to picking up one new fruit and/or veggie and try it out! It may not be your favorite, but what if—just *what if*—you LOVE it? Expanding your palate to include nutrient-dense foods to work *with* and *for* you is an incredible tool to move you closer to your goals and living an abundant life.

Alfalfa Sprouts – These are a member of the pea family, which actually makes them a legume. These seemingly simple sprouts pack quite a nutritional punch, though! Calcium, magnesium, folate, manganese, phosphorus, potassium, sodium, zinc, and vitamins A, B complex, C, E, and K.

Apples – These superstars are a great source of pectin and fiber. They're a wonderful source of vitamins A and C. They also contain calcium, iron, potassium, and phosphorus.

Apricots – This magical fruit is loaded with beta-carotene and fiber, as well as many plant antioxidants. They are a great source of vitamins A (pro-form carotenoids) and C, making them a guilt-free sweet addition to your juice!

Asparagus – Considered an alkaline food, this is also a surprisingly great source of protein, while low in calories and carbs. It's an awesome source of potassium, folate, vitamins A, C, and K, with hints of vitamin B too!

Beets – With more iron than spinach, beets are a great source of vitamins A, B_1, B_2, B_6, and C. They're also a powerhouse full of calcium, magnesium, copper, sodium, and iron.

Bell Peppers – The stronger the color of the pepper, the higher amount of antioxidant properties it contains. This veggie contains more vitamin C in one small pepper than any citrus fruit! Each color pepper contains different phytochemicals, so be sure to mix it up!

Blueberries – Loaded with flavanoids, vitamins B_2, C, and E, fiber, and manganese, these beautiful blues are great for fighting inflammation and supporting a healthy immune system.

Bok Choy – This versatile veggie is a great source of protein, dietary fiber, and almost all the essential vitamins and minerals

Broccoli – Known as a huge disease fighter due to its impressive resume of antioxidants (like quercetin, glutathione, and beta-carotene), it's also rich in vitamin C, A, K, E, B_6, calcium, folate, potassium, and magnesium.

Brussels Sprouts – Great source of vitamins A, C, and E, with moderate amounts of B vitamins. Rich in minerals and phytochemicals, it's also surprisingly a good source of omega-3s and protein!

Cabbage – Containing high levels of calcium, iron, iodine, potassium, sulfur, and phosphorus, it is also loaded with vitamins A, B_1, B_2, B_6, C, E, K, and folate. This versatile veggie is a rich source of a number of phytonutrients too!

Carrots – These are an awesome source of pro-vitamin A, vitamins C, D, E, K, B_1, and B_6. Also rich with biotin, potassium, calcium, magnesium, phosphorus, organic sodium, and some trace minerals, as well as phytonutrients (nature's little disease fighters).

Cantaloupe – A great source of beta-carotene, vitamin C, folic acid, potassium, and dietary fiber, this melon also contains high levels of B vitamins and antioxidants!

Cauliflower – The color varieties contain more phytonutrients. Either way, this veggie is a great source of vitamins B and C.

Cayenne – This spice helps stimulate circulation and neutralize acidity. It's great for digestion, contains anti-inflammatory properties, and is helpful for detoxification.

Celery – Celery leaves contain an abundance of vitamin A. The stems are an excellent source of vitamins B_1, B_2, B_6, and C with rich supplies of potassium, folate, calcium, magnesium, iron, phosphorus, sodium, and plenty essential amino acids.

Chard (Swiss) – This leafy green is a nutritional powerhouse! It's an excellent source of vitamins K, A, and C, as well as a good source of magnesium, potassium, iron, and dietary fiber.

Cherries – These sweet treats provide a ton of antioxidant support, help reduce inflammation, and contain cancer-preventing compounds.

Cilantro – Known for its healing properties—antioxidants and phytonutrients—cilantro is a great source of vitamins A, C, K, and small amounts of B. It also has a good amount of potassium and calcium.

Collard Greens – This leafy green is a nutrient-powerhouse, containing vitamin A and an abundance of B vitamins. Collards also contain high levels of vitamin C and K, as well as folate, calcium, magnesium, and phytonutrients.

Cranberries – Many different studies show this fruit to be one the biggest promoters of antioxidant properties, along with phytonutrients and vitamins A, C, and E, even trace minerals. They also contain B vitamins, folate, and iron.

Cucumber – This veggie contains about 96 percent water, making it a great base for your juice as well as hydration! Its skin is rich in vitamin A, while the whole veggie is a great source of antioxidants and alkaline forming minerals.

Dandelion Greens – A fantastic source of calcium and iron, they're loaded with antioxidants and are a powerful detoxifier! They contain more protein than spinach (per serving) and a lot of minerals!

Fennel – Rich in vitamins A, C, and many of the B's, it's also an excellent source of fiber and essential minerals such as calcium, iron, and copper.

Garlic – Containing amino acids, phytochemicals, and more than twelve types of antioxidants, garlic is also an amazing source of vitamins A, C, and B complex. It's a known anti-inflammatory agent and disease fighter too!

Ginger – Like garlic, ginger is also said to contain more than twelve types of antioxidants, making it a powerful disease fighter. This herb is anti-inflammatory and contains essential oils, protein, calcium, iron, vitamin C, folate, and more! I personally LOVE ginger and eat it daily!

Grapefruit – Of course, we know this is a great source of vitamin C, but don't forget the other important factors included! Like vitamins A, B complex, E, and K. They're also are also packed with minerals and phytonutrients to help fight disease.

Grapes – These little gems include high amounts of vitamins A, B_1, B_2, B_6, and C. They're also loaded with flavanoids—the darker the fruit, the richer in flavanoids! They're full of minerals, such as calcium, copper, iron, magnesium, phosphorus, potassium, and sulfur. Their skins are loaded with phytonutrients, while their seeds are a great source of flavonol antioxidants.

Guava – Packed with a ton of vitamin C (four times more than an orange), vitamin A (ten times more than a lemon), and fiber, this fruit also contains important nutrients like B_2, E, calcium, copper, folate, iron, and potassium.

Habanero Peppers – They are part of the Capsicum family, so the benefits are the same as bell peppers with a good amount of capsaicin, great for digestion and detoxification.

Honeydew Melons – With a high water content, potassium, vitamin C, and copper, they are great for the skin and aiding in collagen production for tissue repair.

Jalapeno Pepper – Like its buddy the habanero, jalapenos contain capsaicin (great for detox and digestion), as well as anti-inflammatory properties.

Jicama – Rich in vitamins A, C, K, and many of the B's, it's great for alkalizing the blood due to its sodium and potassium levels.

Kale – This veggie actually contains a pretty good amount of omega-3 along with iron, potassium, copper calcium, and vitamins C, E, K, B_1, and B_2. It's also a great source of flavanoids and contains anticancer properties.

Kiwi – It may be small, but this fruit has more vitamin C than lemons or oranges! It's also a great source of vitamins A and E, potassium, copper, folate, magnesium, calcium, fiber, and iron.

Lemon – It's an excellent source of vitamin C, B_6, potassium, folate, flavanoids, and the powerful phytochemical limonene.

Lettuce – The darker the leaves, the higher the nutrient content, including chlorophyll. Lettuce is upwards of 90 percent water content, making it great for hydration. It's a great source of fiber and minerals, antioxidants and vitamins, such as A, C, E, K, folate, and B complex.

Lime – An amazing source of calcium and folate, lime is great for women's health.

Mango – With high levels of fiber, pectin, and vitamin C and vitamin A, this sweet fruit is great for alkalizing the body.

Mint – Great for digestion and abundant in vitamins, minerals, and nutrients, mint is a fragrant and tasty addition to juices, smoothies, and dishes alike!

Mustard Greens – Loaded with phytonutrients, this leafy green is a good source of vitamins A and K, fiber, essential minerals, and a moderate source of B complex.

Orange – Just orange orange provides almost 100 percent of the recommended daily dietary intake for vitamin C! Oranges are also a great source of fiber, vitamins A and C, amino acids, potassium, zinc, iron, folate, and calcium.

Parsley – Parsley provides nature's best carotenoids and is a nutrition powerhouse of a few known anticancer and anti-inflammatory phytonutrients and flavonoids. This plant is rich with chlorophyll, vitamins A, B, C, K, folate, and iron. It has a high beneficial mineral content as well.

Papaya – This fruit is so good for digestion, due to the proteolytic enzyme known as papain. In fact, it's so powerful that it's said to digest two hundred times its own weight in protein. It helps our body assimilate and digest the maximum amount of nutrients from our food. Loaded with antioxidants and vitamins A, C, and B, this superstar should be in everyone's diet.

Peaches – Peaches are a good source of antioxidants, they are a moderate source of pro-vitamins, and they are rich in vital minerals such as potassium and iron.

Pear – Pears contain vitamins A, B_1, B_2, C, E, folate, and niacin. They are also a great source of potassium and copper!

Pineapple – An excellent source of C and B_1, it's a great source of potassium, manganese, copper, beta-carotene, fiber, and iron.

Pomegranate – Super high in antioxidants, this fruit contains vitamins B and C, calcium, and phosphorus.

Radish – This often overlooked veggie is rich in vitamins C and B. It is also an excellent source of potassium, calcium, iron, copper, sulfur, phosphorous, and fiber. Radish leaves contain almost six times more vitamin C than the root and they are an amazing source of calcium.

Raspberries – Full of antioxidant and anti-inflammatory benefits, raspberries are a great source of vitamin C.

Spinach – A great source of chlorophyll, spinach is an excellent source of vitamins A, B complex, C, E, K, iron, magnesium, iodine, trace minerals, and amino acids. Its alkalizing properties help with the support of a balanced pH in the body!

Strawberries – Antioxidant-rich, these berries are also a good source of vitamins C and E and beta-carotene.

String Beans – A good source of copper, vitamin B_1, calcium, potassium, phosphorus, vitamin A, protein, iron, vitamin B_6, and vitamin E, string beans are loaded with minerals.

Tomato – Chock-full of vitamins, minerals, and phytonutrients, they are a great source of vitamins C, B_6, and K, beta-carotene, biotin, niacin, potassium, phosphorous, calcium, iron, zinc, and selenium.

Watercress – Watercress is rich in fiber, antioxidants, vitamin C, beta-carotene, folate, potassium, calcium, phosphorous, and iron. It's also a good source of iodine as well.

FACT: This overlooked green contains more calcium than milk and more iron than spinach.

Watermelon – Due to their super-high water content, this sweet summer fruit is excellent for hydration! It's rich in beta-carotene, folate, and vitamin C and a good source of many B vitamins. Watermelon is also loaded with essential minerals and antioxidants.

What Should You Do First?

L ose the old mentality of eating animal protein, dairy, and pasta at every meal. Eating a sensible diet loaded in fruits and vegetables is a much healthier option. When you begin juicing, it does so much more for you than you could ever imagine.

Eating an abundance of uncooked live foods flushes your body of all the unwanted toxic chemicals that are in your body. It leaves you feeling refreshed and rejuvenated and with a much greater sense of peace and well-being. If you have ever done yoga or gotten a back massage, the rejuvenated feeling you have afterward is similar to the effects of consuming a cup of fresh juice. Seriously.

The pure foods give your skin a healthy glow. Radiant, some say. The pure, live food also makes you smell cleaner, leaving you with naturally fresh breath. Sickly people with low immune systems usually report back to me with greater immune function and are in better shape after making juicing a regular part of their life. Getting sick is a thing of the past. One of the great things that I've found while juicing is that my mind is now in control of my body and feeds it only what is necessary for the life of the trillions of cells in my body.

Bonus Video: Immune Boosting Shot

(youtube.com/watch?v=2Hfq3x0MHEY)

Sometimes, if my joints are sore from lifting, I'll have a certain juice (that can be found in this book) and my pains will go away. If my nose is plugged up from allergies and sinus pressure, I am now the holder of a secret juice recipe that will knock that symptom's socks off, getting my sinuses back in working order. If I feel like I'm coming down with a cold, there are several juices that will give me all the immunity I need to push it out, making the illness powerless.

There is so much more that juice can do for you. Research points to certain types of vitamins and minerals in vegetables to be a great preventative measure for many deadly diseases. I'm therefore convinced that fresh vegetable juice is the answer to many of America's health problems. If you're overweight, juice. If you're tired, juice. If you've lost your shine, juice. You get my point.

The only thing you need to get started is a juicer.

Transformation Story

"Today starts week 3 of my juicing and clean eating program . . . I am down 16 pounds and feeling fabulous! I have not had sugar, gluten or dairy in 2 weeks and not missing them at all! I am sleeping through the night and waking up rested! I love this program and the fact that I am eating real food . . . nothing processed!"

—Jill S.

Fruit Juice AND Veggie Juice

The recipes are the "juice" of this book. They are all meant to be mixed and matched. The way I like my juice may be completely different than the way you like your juice. Plus, I've been juicing for a while now, so I'll double up on a lot of the recipes. My advice for you is to experiment, find what you like and enjoy it daily (or as often as possible).

There are some fundamental base mixtures that you can add to any veggie juice. There are also some things with which you'll want to proceed with caution (which are discussed later). Also, just because you are missing one ingredient doesn't mean you should run to the store or not drink the juice with whatever ingredients you have on hand. Juice it up anyway; you might surprise yourself.

Green Juices

Green juices are my go-to; my body just loves green drinks. You want to be careful in the beginning, though. If you are not used to the greens, you could experience some gastric pain. Try mixing your green drinks with apples, cucumbers, celery, or carrots at first.

You can juice (almost) anything green. Cucumbers and celery naturally give more juice than a lot of the leafy or cruciferous vegetables—like broccoli, for example. It's always a good idea to make three-quarters of the cup a watery base by using cucumber or celery and then the rest could be spinach, collard greens, cabbage, or beets. This will be the easiest for your digestion at first. Eventually, your body will become used to the veggies and you will be able to drink an entire glass of spinach juice with no problems.

Fruit and Veggies Don't Always Mix

With a few exceptions, like apples, lemons, and the occasional orange, it's best not to mix your fruits and veggies too much. The fruit will ferment and become much more difficult to break down. For example, what would normally take thirty minutes to process in your body will take up to three hours to process. It's even worse when you have fruit along with grains or meat. This expands digestion time from three hours to eight, which is not good on anybody's system.

To read more transformation stories like the ones in this book, you can find those here: fitlifevip.com/transformationcoaching

From some of our coaches...

"I have just completed my first 90 days of coaching and must say it was an exhilarating event! Taking all the information I learned over the past two years of juicing, learning and participating in all the challenges, it was great to have the opportunity to help others achieve their dreams and goals like I had.

"Not only did I get the chance to encourage others, it made my life move to a new level of appreciation for the ability to help others. Passing the knowledge on and helping men and women achieve a healthy lifestyle is very uplifting and has given me a new respect for myself.

"Coaching enabled me to confirm what I have learned and keeps me focusing on the healthy aspects of my life and those around me. I have learned to not only love the new healthy me, but am encouraging everyone I know to look at how their lives can be improved and reach their transformation goals."

—Coach Linda

"I had no idea what a journey I was beginning when I joined the FitLife Group Coaching program in July 2014. I was about 85 lbs overweight, trying to overcome grief and learning to do life alone. I had no zest for life, no direction and no idea how to move forward.

"I joined the program to lose weight and at this writing, I have lost 71 lbs. But more importantly, I am living an abundant life because of all this journey has given me. My mind is clear, my heart is full, my body is thriving and I know life is limitless.

"Becoming a FitLife Certified Transformation Coach was a continuation of the journey for me. It is so thrilling to walk alongside others as they transform their bodies, and realize their dreams. As a coach, I'm living my dream every day and I invite everyone to join the journey!"

—Coach Lynne

FRUIT JUICES

Recipe Time

1) Kick a Virus

An apple a day keeps the doctor away. There is truth to this in that the nutrients found in apples have been known to boost immune function. This is one of my favorite juices to have in the morning and it will keep you from getting ill.

- 2 apples
- 1 orange

Peel the orange and cut the seeds out of the apple; they are not good for you. If the apples are not organic, don't even bother— they are loaded with chemicals. Get organic. It will cost you a little more, but the benefits are entirely worth it.

2) The Arouser

Skip the pills for erectile dysfunction and start juicing this. You will notice a *BIG* difference. Try adding a little apple juice for more of a complex taste.

- 2 bunches black grapes
- 1-inch piece ginger
- 4 strawberries, hulled
- ½ cup pitted black cherries

Many of the fruits and vegetables in these recipes will assist you in the bedroom because they enhance your circulatory system. If the blood is pumping, your sexual organs should be working as well. Some fruits and vegetables assist more than others and this happens to be a combination that tastes great—and works great too!

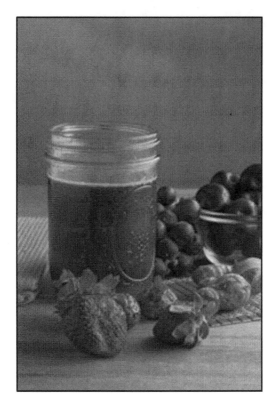

3) Aches, Pains, and Sinus Drains

Simple, but amazing. Pineapple juice will cure aches and pains in your body. Sometimes I'll come back from the gym and rock out some APSD juice. If it's not organic, get rid of the skin. Cut the pineapple into long strips and juice it up. Make sure you wash the outside of the pineapple before you begin. Sometimes, when cutting, you can drag the nasty toxins inside to the meat of the pineapple.

- 1 whole pineapple (if organic, you can juice the skin; if not, cut it off)

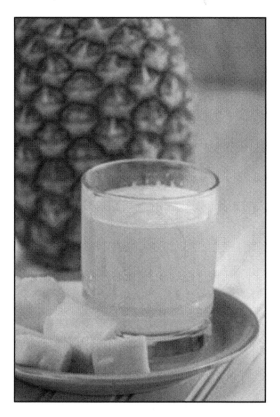

4) Cantaloupe Juice

Cantaloupe supplies the body with beta-carotene and aids in digestion. Beta-carotene is the only source of carotene that can be turned into vitamin A by the body. Vitamin A is absolutely critical to your health, assisting in your eyesight, bone growth, cell reproduction, and cell division. Vitamin A also helps maintain healthy skin and mucus membranes that defend against bacteria and viruses and helps regulate the immune system.

- ½ cantaloupe

Cut the skin off and make the pieces small enough to pop in the juicer. Make sure when cutting the melon that you wash the skin first; again, you don't want to drag the nasties inside the melon.

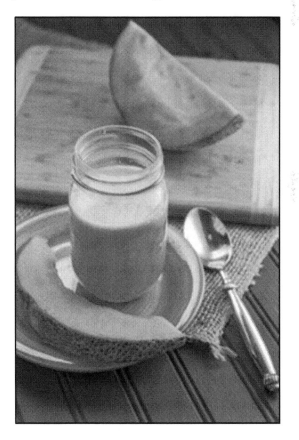

5) The Einstein

Grapefruit juice is great for controlling insulin levels on cheat days. It will give you energy as well as massive amounts of focus. This is a great pre-workout drink in the morning. I personally love grapefruit; it's my favorite fruit. It's low in carbs and calories and can speed up your metabolism.

- 1 grapefruit (if organic, you can juice the skin; if not, cut it off)

6) Pimp Juice

Feel like impressing your lady friend on a warm summer evening?

- 4 apricots
- 1 bunch red grapes, preferably organic, with stems
- 1 pear

Take the pits out of the apricots and cut the pear in half. Throw it in the juicer and turn on the music. It's about to go down.

7) R.E.L.A.X.

This juice always seems to bring me peace after a long day at work. It's also great for hydration, aches, and pains.

- 2 (1-inch) pineapple rounds, preferably organic
- 2 celery stalks

If not organic, skin the pineapple.

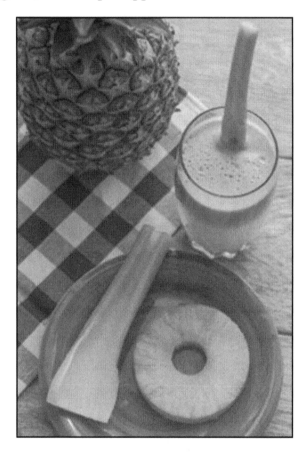

8) Cantaloupe Apple

This supplies the body with a lot of beta-carotene, which is a disease-fighting substance. It also aids in digestion. The apple adds a great flavor, along with additional health benefits

- ¼ full-size melon
- 1 apple

9) Immunity Plus (Plus)

This drink will boost your immune system faster than you can say, "I am a super hero!" Cranberries are great for your GI tract and for ridding your body of unwanted bacteria.

- 3 apples
- 1 cup cranberries

Cut the seeds out of the apple (use organic apples only). Put the rest of the fruit in the juicer.

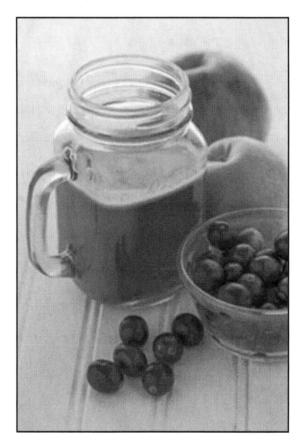

10) Holistic Holiday Ginger Blast

This is a great juice to make for your guests and visitors around the holidays. Want to make sure your kids come home to visit you every year? Apples have a lot of great natural sugar and they aid digestion. Make this juice and seal the deal.

- 3 apples
- 2 bunches grapes
- 1 tiny piece ginger
- 1 lemon

Peel the lemon and apples if they are not organic and get rid of the grape stems if not organic. Wash well.

11) Laugh Attack Juice

I was sitting at the kitchen table with a dear friend and this juice forced us to go into a fit of laughter for no reason. Try it and laugh yourself silly.

- 1 cup cranberries
- 1 bunch green grapes, preferably organic, with stems
- 1 (1-inch) pineapple round

If the grapes are not organic, remove the stems. If the pineapple is not organic, same deal; remove the rind.

Laughing can burn calories! It increases your T-cells and globulins, which aid in immune system function. It also decreases your stress hormones (cortisol, adrenaline, and DOPAC). When we laugh, our body responds positively.

12) Brain Juice

I don't know what it is about this juice, but when I drink it I feel like my mental acuity spikes instantly. It's probably the B_6 in the broccoli that gets my mind so revved up!

- 1 broccoli shoot and floret, diced
- 1 cucumber
- 1 lemon
- ½ carrot

Dice the broccoli up so that it fits in the juicer. Peel the lemon if it is not organic.

13) Attack the Day

Nothing gives me more energy in the morning than some freshly squeezed, high-quality orange juice. If you bought your juicer only for oranges, you made a wise decision. Once you try this you will NEVER want store-bought OJ again!

- 3 oranges

If they are not organic, make sure you peel them. If they are organic, just throw them in the juicer. Eating a whole orange can provide you with an abundance of fiber. Sometimes I eat the orange as I would an apple.

One orange has over 170 phytonutrients and more than 60 flavonoids, many of which have been shown to have anti-inflammatory, antitumor, and blood clot-inhibiting properties, as well as strong antioxidant effects.

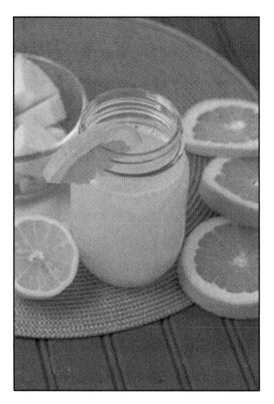

14) Spartacus Juice

This is a great juice to drink before going into battle—or going to the gym. Whichever. With all of the vitamins of the orange and the insulin controls of the grapefruit, you can't go wrong drinking this pre-workout. It gives me loads of energy for battling against the evil bench press descending from Capua.

- 1 orange
- ¼ grapefruit
- 1 lemon

If all your fruit is organic, leave the skin. If not, cut it off and process in the juicer.

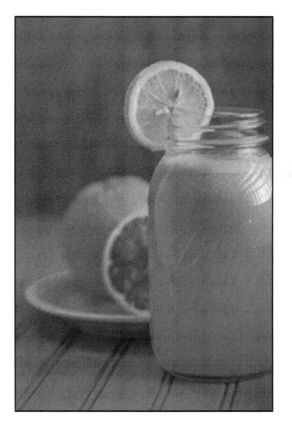

15) Love Juice

If love had a flavor, this would be it. This has an unimaginable contrast between the apple, mango, and the pear. It's great for a dessert juice or in the morning after sleeping in. You owe it to yourself to try it.

- 2 apples
- 1 pear
- ¼ mango
- 3 strawberries

Drink it slowly and offer gratitude for the day. Peel the mango and anything else that is not organic. Juice the mango first and the strawberries last to turn this into a tasty sunrise of love and adoration for the day.

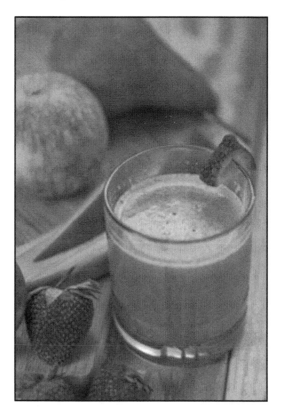

16) Purple Passion Juice

This one is fun to make because of the pomegranate. It's perfect for a warm summer day. Put it on ice and give a glass to your neighbor. Who knows, maybe they will start mowing your lawn for you.

- ½ cup pomegranate
- 1 apple
- 1 bunch purple grapes (take the stems off if not organic)

Dice the pomegranate into pieces. If the juice is a little too bitter, take the seeds out.

Pomegranate juice is a rich source of sodium and also contains a good amount of riboflavin, thiamine, niacin, Vitamin C, calcium and phosphorous—a very powerful antioxidant.

17) Fruit Cocktail

This is a great-tasting juice that is great for cookouts and family get-togethers. If it's a hot summer day, you could always throw the fruit in a blender with some ice. Amazing!

- 1 orange
- ½ lime with skin
- ¼ cup blueberries
- 1 cup sparkling mineral water

Peel the orange to rid the drink of the bitterness and cut the lime in half so the juicer can handle it. If it is not organic, peel it. Pour the juice and add the sparkling water. Add lime or orange to garnish it.

18) Real Gatorade

This is a great drink to quench thirst during a long workout or run. Water is always the best, but most fruit is up to 60 percent water.

- 1 orange
- 1 lime
- 1 cup water

This drink will hydrate you and give you some much-needed vitamin C to ward off colds and keep you healthy. Put this on ice if it is hot outside.

I was talking to one of the vendors at a local farmers' market and they told me it is best to eat the fruits that are in season if you are trying to stay hydrated. The in-season fruit will have less packaging time and will offer the best hydrating benefits. It's also the least expensive! Makes sense.

19) Miss Georgia Juice

Everyone loves a great-tasting, supple peach. This drink tastes amazing! Peaches are a great source in vitamin A, magnesium, and potassium. Grab yourself a glass of this and smile.

- 1 orange
- 1 peach
- ¼ cup mineral water
- 1 orange slice, to make it look cool

Pit the peach. Add the orange. Once you have your juice, add the mineral water and smile. I don't know why, but this drink makes me smile—probably because it's also good for your teeth.

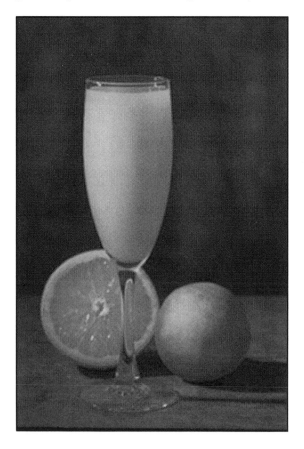

20) Ginger Ginger Ginger (or Ginger³)

Let me introduce you to my good friend, Ginger. You have to start slow with her or she will bite you. She's a spicy one! She is great for pressing out toxins from your body and adding a little flair. Also great for your immune system and combating excess inflammation in your body.

- 2 apples
- 1 orange
- 1 knob ginger

Start this juice with the apple and end with the apple. This will press the rest of the ginger out of the juicer. Peel the orange and apple if they are not organic.

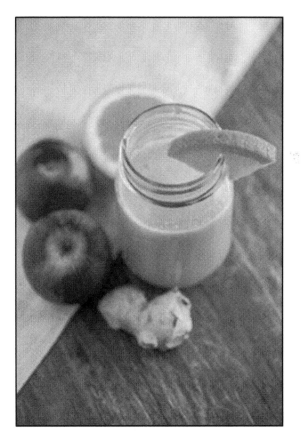

21) Grapple Punch

This juice has a little punch to it that you will love.

- 1 bunch green grapes
- 1 pineapple rind
- 1 lemon (with skin, if organic)
- 1 cup mineral water

This is a great juice for you and the whole family. Remove the skin from the pineapple and the lemon if they are not organic. Put mineral water in. Why mineral water? Most water has to be processed and during this processing it loses minerals. Mineral water, conversely, is usually found in a mineral-rich water source and has many health benefits.

22) Mountain "Drew"

This won't make you crash like the other green stuff. Sweet and sour, it's like drinking candy.

- 12 ounces of honeydew melon (approximately ¼ of the melon)
- ½ lime, with skin

Cut the honeydew into strips. Slice up the lime. Process the fruit all together.

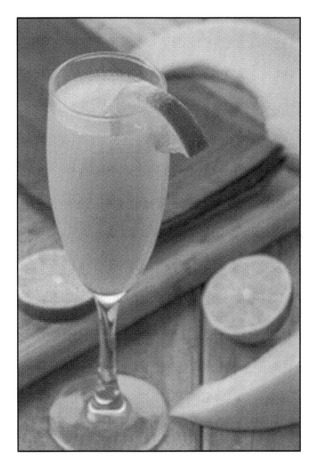

23) California Love

Nothing can describe the flavor of California better than the lusciously passionate pineapple and the sexy, succulent strawberries. Put these two together and you have California in a cup. Don't believe me? Try it. I dare you.

- 1 pineapple round
- 8–10 strawberries

If the pineapple is not organic, remove the skin. Process the fruit in the juicer. Enjoy the taste of California. If you don't live in California and would like to, imagine yourself on the beach while sipping on this cup of California Koolaid in hand.

24) Kiwi Kick Myself Silly

This one is like a karate convention in your mouth. The flavors jump-kick you in the tongue as you slurp down this bad boy.

- 1 bunch green grapes
- 3 kiwis
- 1 orange
- 3 strawberries

Mmmmm . . . so good! What more can I say? Make sure you peel your fruit if it is not organic (excluding the strawberries).

FACT: Laughter triggers the release of endorphins, the body's natural feel-good chemicals. Endorphins promote an overall sense of well-being and can even temporarily relieve pain.

25) Slap Happy Sammy

This drink will make you happy beyond measure. There is something about a mango that brings a sense of well-being into your life. Imagine for a moment the taste of the mango. Smiling yet?

- 1 mango
- 3 strawberries
- ½ lemon, with skin
- 1 apple

Remove the skin from the mango, peel it in half, and remove the pit. Remove the skin on the apple if it is not organic. When you drink this, think back to a memory or a time where you felt really good about your life. Maybe there was a certain someone or something. Focus on that and enjoy!

26) Tenacious Titillating Tampa Juice

When I first moved from Michigan to Florida, I thought I'd died and gone to heaven. Nothing against Michigan, it's a great place. It just didn't have fields upon fields of tropical fruit, like Tampa.

- 2 oranges
- ¼ pineapple, sliced lengthwise

Make sure to peel the orange and the pineapple, if they are not organic. Cut the orange so it can fit in your juicer.

27) Sweet and Sour Patch Morning

Enjoy the sweet flavor of the pineapple and the sour of the grapefruit.

- 1 pineapple round
- 1 grapefruit

This drink will help kick-start your day and give you massive amounts of energy for a morning workout. Try it and let me know how it works.

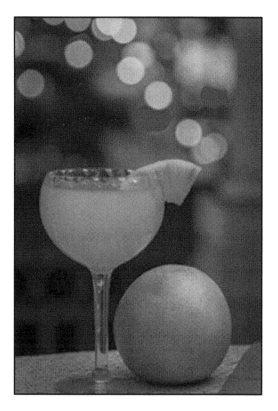

28) Zen Zinger

This is the juice of peace and tranquility. If you are experiencing any problems in your relationships, drink this juice and know that it will work out how it's supposed to.

- 2 Golden Delicious sweet apples
- 1–2-inch knob fresh ginger
- 3 kiwis
- Piece of sage, for garnish

Peel the fruit if any of it isn't organic. Start with an apple and end with an apple. When you drink this juice really center on that person who brings you a great deal of love in your life. Shift your awareness to someone who you are having trouble with and see that same type of love in that other person. Blanket them with love.

29) Fist Pumpin' Party Time!

Turn the music up and start dancing! This juice is guaranteed to put a little toot in your booty. (I don't really know what that means, but run with it anyway.)

- 1 pineapple round
- 1 orange
- ½ lemon, with skin

If the pineapple is not organic, remove and discard the skin. Same goes for the orange and lemon, or wash it really well.

30) Passion Juice

Whether you want to impress your significant other or just love yourself, try this juice on for size. It will make your taste buds stand up and start hugging each other like crazed hippies.

- 1 pineapple round
- 1 bunch grapes
- 8 strawberries, hulled
- ½ lemon
- Piece of strawberry, for garnish

Peel the pineapple if it is not organic. Remove the stems from the grapes and cut the lemon in half.

31) Papple Juice

This is a combination of two of my favorite fruits—apple and pear. Yum! This is a great juice to drink while eating raw, organic cheese (hormone- and antibiotic-free).

- 2 apples
- 1 pear

Peel both if they are not organic and cut the seeds out of the apple. Enjoy this over ice on a warm summer day.

32) Pink Panther Flush

This is another sweet and sour classic of mine. Great before the gym or if you just want a little hop in your step. This juice will help control your insulin levels while getting your sugar from the apples and using the ginger to press out toxins. Brilliant!

- 2 apples
- ½ grapefruit
- 1 knuckle fresh ginger

Make sure you peel the apples if they are not organic. Put an apple in first and last.

33) San Francisco Fog Basher

This is a great drink in the morning to get your heart pumping and your mind awake. If you are experiencing lack of focus, this is a fantastic drink. The lemon will help alkalize your body as well.

- 2 apples
- 8 strawberries
- 1 lemon

Peel the apples if they are not organic. Cut the seeds out from the apple core as well. Wash your lemon with some veggie wash or soak it in grapefruit juice and water.

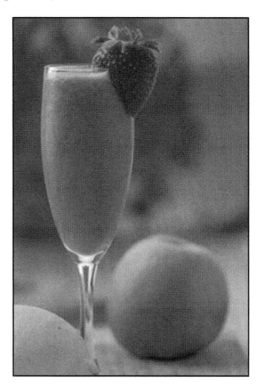

34) Drew Juice

This is my favorite fruit juice. First of all, I love the flavor of apple juice. And when the ginger is added, it gives it an amazing kick. Of course, I'm the guy who would chew on ginger if it were lying around. This is a great one for cold prevention, as well.

- 4 apples
- 1 ginger piece

Try this juice out and you will know what I'm talking about. Make sure you peel your apple if it is not organic and get rid of the seeds in the core.

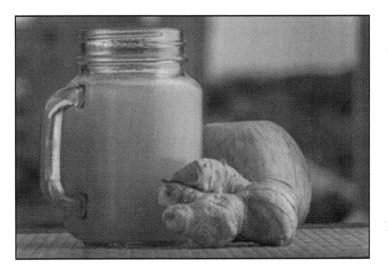

35) Lucy Juice

I have a friend and this is her absolute all-time favorite. It's a simple mix and can be mixed with champagne. (That's the way she likes it.)

- 1 bunch purple grapes
- 8 strawberries

Get rid of the stems if the grapes are not organic. Pour a little champagne on top to turn this into a party drink or if you need a little hair-o'-the-dog.

36) Sunrise Juice

There's nothing more magnificent or captivating than waking up every morning to catch a good sunrise. I've been in this discipline for years and many times I like to have this type of juice accompany me.

- 2 apples
- 4 strawberries
- 1 lemon
- 1 handful cherries (from Michigan if you can)

Cut the skin off the apple if it is not organic and wash the rest of your fruit. If you are fortunate enough to have a good view of the sun in the morning, drink this to salute it and give thanks to the sun for providing you with light and warmth throughout the day.

37) Watermelon Kidney Flush

This is a great juice to detoxify your kidneys and leave you feeling refreshed and rejuvenated. Very sugar-based, so you might want to do one part water to one part juice.

- ½ baby watermelon

Dice up the watermelon to fit in the juicer. Make sure you wash the skin well. This is where the majority of the nutrients are held.

38) Lemme Eat the Apple

- 2 apples
- 1 lemon
- 1-inch slice ginger

If the apples are organic, juice them with their skins on. The skin is the most abundant area of the apple for flavonoid content. This will produce cloudy but more nutritious (and still delicious) apple juice recipes. This healthy juicer recipe also makes a great remedy for colds. Peel the lemon if it is not organic.

39) Berry Medley

- 2 cups strawberries
- 2 cups blueberries
- 1 ½ cups raspberries

Berries are among the quickest and easiest of fruits to juice. The only prepping they need is a quick rinse. Strawberries are a small exception, as they will need their tops removed before juicing.

40) Breakfast Bounce

This will put a little bounce in your step.

- 3 oranges
- 1 grapefruit

Make sure you peel the oranges and the grapefruit. Place fruit in the juicer and enjoy.

41) Kiwi Blue

This is a classic for anyone who loves a sweet little treat.

- 3 kiwis
- 2 cups blueberries

Peel kiwis, wash berries, juice, enjoy.

Blue fruits, such as the highly esteemed blueberries, contain a wide variety of phytochemicals. Anthocyanins give blueberries their amazing color. Blueberries contain other phytochemicals that can improve memory. They are also a great anti-aging and anti-inflammatory fruit.

42) Fresh Lemonade

If this were sold on the street corner by the neighbor's kid, it would be worth more than a quarter. You really can't beat this recipe.

- 2 or 3 large lemons
- ½ cup water
- 1 apple to sweeten, optional

Peel lemons and cut stem of apple. (Swap out 1 lemon for 1 lime and bingo, you've got limeade). Add ice on those hot days.

43) The Silent Strawberry

Love this combination! The strawberry is subtle and it just sneaks up on you.

- 1/3 cup strawberries
- 1 cup blueberries
- 2 apples

Wash all the ingredients well and juice.

Red fruits, such as strawberries, contain the phytochemical lycopene, which gives them their red color. Lycopene has been shown to help prevent prostate cancer and heart disease.

44) Pear and Kiwi Juice

This is a great energy juice and is high in vitamin C.

- 2 kiwis
- 2 pears

Peel kiwis and remove pear stems. People will really enjoy this juice.

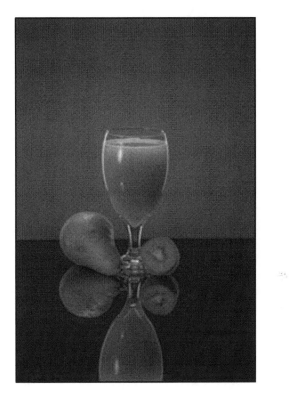

45) Melon Medley

Like melons on a hot summer day, you will enjoy this even more. Tantalize your taste buds with this juice. Don't say I didn't warn you.

- ½ watermelon
- ½ honeydew melon
- ½ cantaloupe

Remove rinds and seeds (except for watermelon seeds). Put contents in the juicer and enjoy.

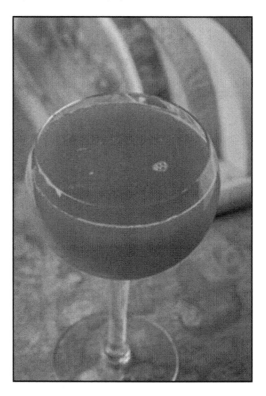

46) Tropical Fruit Juice Recipes

My mother loves this one. She is up in Michigan most of the year, but when she visits me in Florida, I serve this juice.

- 1 orange
- 1 kiwi
- ½ mango
- Sparkling mineral water

Peel all the fruits and pit the mango. Pour the juice in a large glass, fill to the top with sparkling water, and serve.

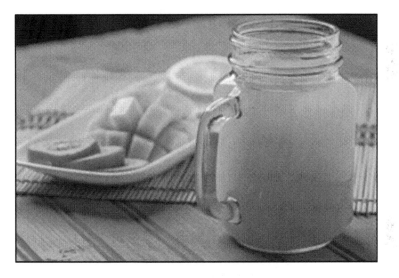

47) Kidney Cleanse

This juice has been proven to clean your kidneys out. Careful on the watermelon; it is really sweet.

- 2 apples
- 3 ½ watermelon pieces with rind (about 1-inch pieces)

Wash your fruit. Even slicing a melon that is non-organic can pull the toxins from the outside in. Cut the apples into narrow wedges and juice with the watermelon pieces. Juice and enjoy healthy kidneys.

48) The Pain Reducer

This juice will help relieve you from aches and pains.

- 1 lemon
- 1 orange
- 2 hard pears
- 2 apples

Peel lemon and orange, remove pear and apple stems, and juice.

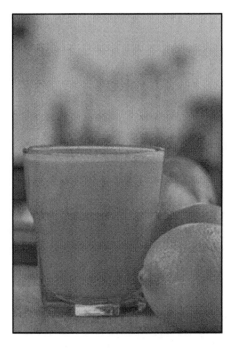

Bonus Video: Get Rid of Joint Pain
youtube.com/watch?v=LYM8bSzctrs

49) S² (Supreme Splendid)

Once this juice hits your lips the word "splendid" will come out of your mouth. I promise.

- 1 orange, peeled and sectioned
- 1 cup fresh pineapple, cubed, skin removed
- 5 strawberries

Peel orange and pineapple and remove the tops from the strawberries. Process the fruit in a juicer and serve. You are going to love this juice.

50) Five-Star Tropical Lineup

Nothing says the tropics like this juice. The combination of guava and mango is amazing. Remember, I'm not neglecting anything from the rest of this all-star cast. You are going to become addicted to this juice.

- 1 mango
- 1 large orange
- 1 pineapple slice
- 1 papaya
- 1 guava

Peel and remove all pits and seeds. This is another favorite juice recipe of mine. Awesome on a hot day with ice!

VEGETABLE JUICES

Recipe Time

This is where the start of lifelong health and anti-aging begins. I hope you are as excited as I am. Fruit juices are great for overall health and well-being, but nothing says, "I'm going to live to be 200!" like an energizing green drink.

Vegetables are the building blocks to life. They supply your body with all of the necessary vitamins and minerals necessary for energy, vitality, and LIFE. Did you know that there is actually more protein in most leafy greens—like spinach and collard greens—than there is in a steak? These greens are 45 percent protein. However, you have to eat a lot of spinach to get the same amount that is in that piece of animal flesh. Why not juice it instead? The veggies, not the meat. :) Plus, the juice actually tastes better! It's fresh and vibrant. You can taste the life force energy as it moves throughout your body.

Some of these recipes will recommend a little bit of fruit for taste, although it's not necessary. These are my recipes after many wins and an occasional loss here or there. I remember a few juices that no one would drink!

Most of these juices will be absolutely delicious, and if by chance you don't like a recipe and want to alter it, feel free. This book is to help get you started and give you some ideas. Get creative. Experiment. Share with your loved ones.

Bonus Video: Anti-Aging Juice Recipe:
youtube.com/watch?v=Yw-9suOdGTU

1) Recharge Your Alkaline Battery

Do you have gas in your pants? Feel tired or acidic? Maybe you've had one too many coffees today? This juice will help you bounce back quickly.

- 1 handful red cabbage
- 1 cucumber
- 1 handful spinach
- 1 lemon

Cut the skin off the cucumber if it is not organic; it's good to get rid of the wax they put on it. If you have the option, buy plastic-wrapped, pesticide-free cucumbers. Juice the rest of the veggies as normal.

FACT: Disease cannot live in an alkaline state. Having a balanced pH is important to keep you healthy. Overconsumption of sugar, gluten, grains, dairy, caffeine, alcohol, and animal protein contributes to an acidic environment so be sure to eat plenty of greens to detoxify the body and help rebalance it for optimal health.

2) Anti-Ulcer/Probiotic Juice

Looking to balance your system out? This juice will do it. When the going gets tough, the tough get juicing. There are all kinds of probiotics in this glass of greens. Great drink for clearing free radicals and disease prevention.

- ¼ red cabbage
- 2 handfuls of spinach
- 4 collard green leaves
- 4 celery stalks

Wash all of your veggies and start juicing.

Probiotics are live microorganisms that, when administered in adequate amounts, confer a health benefit on the host. I like to think of probiotics as little bodyguards in my intestinal track. If something nasty comes in, they clean up the mess.

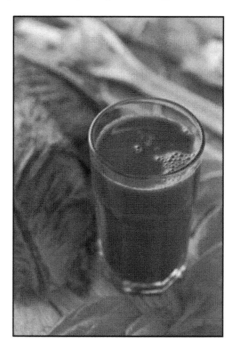

3) Anti-Acne Miracle Skin

This juice has been used to clear the skin from within. It is great for anyone who spends hundreds of dollars per year on late-night infomercial pimple creams.

- 6 carrots
- ½ green bell pepper

Cut the tops off the carrots and bell pepper, rinse, juice, and drink. When drinking this juice, visualize the ingredients providing enough nutrients and energy to rid your body of the toxins causing these blemishes. See them going away. See your skin as clear and glowing. And so it will be.

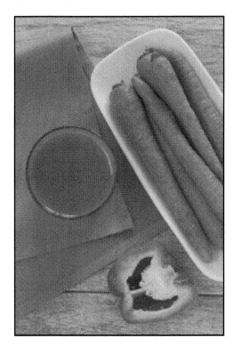

4) Life Regenerator Blood Boost

Drink this juice to purify and give your blood the iron it needs. A 180-gram serving of boiled spinach contains 6.43 milligrams of iron, whereas one 170-gram ground hamburger patty contains, at most, 4.42 milligrams.

- 5 carrots
- 1 handful parsley
- 2 radishes
- 6 spinach leaves
- 4 lettuce leaves
- 1 piece of ginger

Trim the tops of the carrots off and wash all your vegetables. Put them in the juicer and enjoy. Drink this juice slowly. I usually spend 15 minutes drinking a juice like this. "Chew your juice" to really get the most benefit.

Ever wonder why Popeye was so strong? Iron is the main ingredient in hemoglobin, which is found in red blood cells and is responsible for carrying oxygen throughout the body. Without enough iron, the body is unable to produce enough hemoglobin and, as a result, muscles get less oxygen, which reduces the body's energy.

5) Body Purifier

I drink this juice to flush out the necessary toxins and give my heart a boost.

- 2 carrots
- 1 cucumber
- ½ cauliflower
- ½ beet

Cut the top off the carrots and peel the skin off of the cucumber if it is not organic. Many times, if the beet is not organic, the chemicals will be at the base where the beet and the stems connect. Make sure it is clean or cut it off completely.

6) Bone Builder

Strong bones are essential to good health. Many vegetables take on the shape and form of what they are good for in the body. If you look at celery, it looks like your bones. So, as you might guess, celery is the chosen vegetable here.

- 8 celery stalks
- 2 carrots
- 1 bunch parsley
- 1 lemon

Dice the celery up small enough to fit in your juicer (if necessary) and trim the tops off the carrot. Peel them if they are not organic and wash your vegetables.

Diet/nutrition is the key ingredient to great heart health. Adding carrots and cauliflower are two good things you can do, being low in salt and easy to tolerate. Stick to a raw diet as much as possible. This will allow your heart to heal the quickest.

7) Capri Kiddie Juice

When kids won't eat their veggies, it's because they like sweet stuff. So this is your healthy key to sweeten up the green goodness of the broccoli and cucumber.

- 1 broccoli floret
- 1 cucumber
- 2 apples

Just be careful not to give them too much apple juice because they could start running around the house at an accelerated rate. Trim all of the vegetables so they fit in the juicer. Peel them if they are not organic.

8) Simply Green Machine

Green drinks are my favorite and more often I go to this type of juice. Enjoy this one. The parsley is great for eliminating bad breath and body odor.

- 1 cup spinach
- 2 cups kale
- 2 cups parsley
- 1 cucumber
- 3 celery stalks

Add a little garlic and/or ginger if you like. Wash thoroughly and juice.

Parsley is a good source of folic acid, one of the most important B vitamins. It plays a lot of key roles in your body, but chief among them is your cardiovascular health. The flavonoids in parsley have been shown to function as antioxidants that combine with highly reactive oxygen-containing molecules (called oxygen radicals) and help prevent oxygen-based damage to cells.

In addition, extracts from parsley have been used in animal studies to help increase the antioxidant capacity of the blood reducing tumors.

9) Cuke-Apple Zippy

This has a great zip to it. I love ginger in my juices.

- 2 ½ apples
- ½ cucumber
- 1-inch piece of ginger

Remove apple stems and juice everything together.

10) Heaven Sent

You know anything with the word "heaven" in the title has to be amazing. Just try it and tell me what you think.

- 1 cup spinach
- ½ cucumber
- 2 celery stalks, including leaves
- 3 carrots
- ½ apple

Wash everything thoroughly, cut the tops off the carrots, remove apple stem, juice, and enjoy.

11) The Cucapple

Simple yet satisfying, hydrating, and energy-packed.

- ½ cucumber
- 2 apples

Remove the stems from the apples, cut the cucumber in half, and juice. The nice thing about both apples and cucumbers is that you get a lot of juice out of them. This is great when you just need something quick.

12) Parsley Pump Up

This is one of my favorite juices as well. There is nothing like fresh parsley in a juice to clean out your system.

- 1 cup parsley
- ½ apple
- 2 carrots
- 3 celery stalks

Wash all thoroughly, remove apple stem, remove the tops from the carrots, juice, and enjoy!

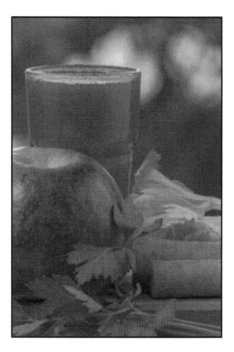

13) Bless My Eyes, for Now I Can See!

Carrots and kale, what more can I say? Did Bugs Bunny ever wear glasses? No. Did he have X-ray vision like Superman? No. Will you have X-ray vision? Probably not.

- 6 carrots
- 1 cup kale

That's right—carrots are great for your eyes! Okay, it's not the actual carrot; it is the beta-carotene that is *in* the carrot. When it is converted to vitamin A in the liver, it is then transformed to rhodopsin, a purple-colored pigment that is used at night to see. Beta-carotene is a powerful antioxidant that aids against macular degeneration, which happens to be the leading cause of blindness in the elderly.

14) Liver Life

Clean your liver and everything else.

- ½ beet, with greens
- 3 apples

Wash all thoroughly, remove apple stems, and put the beet in.

15) Green Juice Recipes Energizer

This one is a real blast, brimming with goodness. It's one of my favorite weight-loss juices as well.

- 2 apples
- ½ cucumber
- ½ lemon, peeled
- ½ cup kale
- ½ cup spinach
- ¼ bunch celery
- ¼ bulb fennel
- 1-inch piece ginger
- ¼ head romaine lettuce

Kale is high in beta-carotene. Kale also has a significant supply of vegetable protein that is amazing for your body. Next time you are at the market, look for kale's healthy but ignored cousins—Swiss chard, mustard greens, and collards.

16) My Memory, Oh My!

This juice will activate your brain to help recall memories from the past. This is great for students who are about to take an exam. The mint is the key.

- 1 cucumber
- 1 carrot
- 1 green apple
- ¼ cup parsley
- ¼ cup mint
- 1 celery stalk
- ½-inch piece fresh ginger
- ½ lemon, peeled

Wash and peel all of your non-organic vegetables. Cut up to fit in the juicer and enjoy.

17) Energizer Bunny

If you are in an energy slump, this is the juice for you. Get ready to turn your nine-volt back on. This juice will get you revved up and ready to face the day.

- 2 carrots
- 1 broccoli floret
- 2 handfuls spinach
- ½ beet
- 1 lemon
- 1 knob fresh ginger

You will love this juice. It's one of my personal favorites. Trim up the carrots so they fit in the juicer. If the lemon is not organic, trim the skin off that as well.

18) Sleep Better Sally

I sometimes drink this juice if I'm having trouble sleeping. It not only helps you sleep, it cleans your system out while you drift off into la-la land. Magnesium and zinc are vitamins that help you slumber. Both spinach and kale are high in magnesium and zinc.

- 2 handfuls spinach
- 4 celery stalks
- 3 kale leaves
- 1 lemon

This is a great natural detox, but I make sure to brush my teeth after this drink and before bed because the lemon has acid in it that is bad for your teeth's enamel. You don't want it sitting on your teeth while you're sleeping.

19) C2L

This juice calms me and gives me focused energy throughout the night. If you've had a long day at the office, but still have a busy night ahead of you and need to get lots of stuff done, this is the juice for you.

- ¼ red cabbage
- 2 carrots
- 1 lemon

Drink this juice slowly so your body absorbs the nutrients. Trim the tops off the carrots and dice them up to fit them in the juicer. I drink this after a long workout and it eliminates a lot of the fatigue I experience.

Cabbage is amazing! It has the ability to aid you in your digestion process. It is also rich in antioxidants and loaded with anti-inflammatory effects.

20) Apple and Cauliflower Juice

Normally I'm not fond of the way cauliflower tastes, but when you release a few magical golden delicious apples into the center of it, you will be very satisfied.

- 3 apples
- ½ cauliflower head

Peel the apple if it is not organic and make sure you wash the cauliflower thoroughly.

21) Carrot and Celery Juice

Celery is a great base juice for any of your mixes. It doesn't hold a lot of flavor but it is amazing for your bones. When you add the carrot to the celery juice, it gives you the flavor you are looking for.

- 6 celery stalks
- 3 carrots

Trim up your veggies so they fit in the juicer; remember to cut the tops off of the carrots and wash thoroughly.

22) The Orange and Green Mohawk

This brightly colored drink is amazing for your digestive tract, and it tastes great too!

- 4 carrots
- ½ beet
- 1 handful parsley

Trim the tops off of the carrots and beet. Wash your veggies.

23) Cauliflower Broccoli Monster

This is a drink that will leave you feeling strong. There is no wonder in it either; there is a ton of phosphorus in both cauliflower and broccoli.

- 3 carrots
- ½ broccoli floret
- ½ cauliflower head

Trim the top off the carrot and dice your veggies up enough to fit in your juicer. Bookend your juice with the carrots to maximize your juice efforts. When drinking this juice, really feel the protein from the broccoli go into your cells.

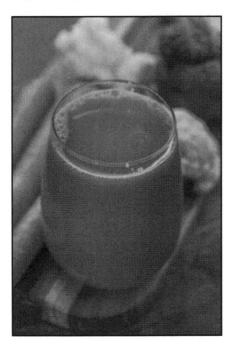

24) The Ripley (Believe It or Not)

This is the juice that could have saved Mr. Ripley's life and has been one of his all-time favorites since he started. It also helps that it doesn't cost an arm and a leg to make.

- 3 apples
- 3 carrots

Peel your apples if they are not organic and remove the seeds. Trim the tops from the carrots and voilà!

25) Lake City Winter Blues

This is a drink that will warm you up and get your blood boiling. It's especially great in my hometown, Lake City, Michigan. What better way to warm up your body functions than by heating them up with some nutritious, bold, and tasty juice. This juice will chase away the winter blues.

- 2 carrots
- ½ beet
- 1 handful parsley
- 1 handful cilantro
- 1 pinch cayenne pepper
- 1 tomato
- 1 cup tonic

Wash all of your vegetables thoroughly. Trim the tops off of the carrots and the beat. Put the parsley and cilantro in toward the middle. Once the juice is complete, add the tonic and you are off. Garnish with a pickle, if you must.

26) Cholesterol Cruncher

This juice will kick your cholesterol to the curb.

- 2 bundles bok choy
- 8 asparagus spears
- 1 apple
- 1-inch piece ginger
- 2 handfuls spinach

Wash all your veggies thoroughly. Dice your apple into pieces, remove the seeds, and peel it if it is not organic. When you drink this juice, imagine your blood cleaning out and getting healthier. This visualization technique will be helpful in the healing process.

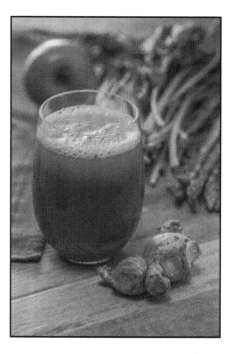

27) Blood Infusion

This is a power-packed drink for your blood and heart. It opens up your circulatory system. Both beetroot and greens are powerful cleansers and builders of the blood.

- ½ beet
- 2 red chard leaves
- 2 carrots
- ½ cucumber
- Dash cayenne

Wash the beets and trim the tops off. Clean the red chard and cut the tops off the carrots. Enjoy the sweet spice of this drink.

28) Carrot Spinach Juice (GI Tract Special)

This juice helps with digestion and is packed with vitamins. Powerful stuff! It goes well with your meal.

- 4 or 5 carrots
- 3 handfuls spinach
- 1 broccoli floret

Trim the tops off of the carrots and wash the spinach.

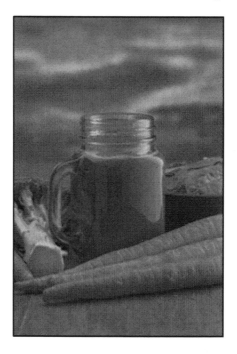

29) Stomach Soother

Any juice containing cabbage soothes the stomach as long as it is mixed with a milder juice.

- ½ cabbage
- 4 carrots
- 2 apples
- 1 piece ginger

Trim the cabbage and carrots so that they can fit in the juicer. Remove the apple seeds.

30) White Eye Juice

Ever wonder why people who eat only raw food have whiter eyes? This is one of my secret juices that will clean your eyes. Normally, when a person's eyes are red, it's due to stress or a stressed out liver. This will detox your liver and get it working for you again.

Start by avoiding alcohol, refined sugar, and trans fat. You want to support your liver as much as possible, allowing it to do its job in detoxing your body and clearing out the clutter.

- 2 collard greens leaves
- 4 carrots
- 2 kale leaves
- 2 mustard green leaves
- 1 lemon

Wash all your vegetables thoroughly. Trim the tops of the carrots. Peel the lemon if it is not organic.

The liver is the largest gland in the body. It eliminates toxic chemicals in your blood. It also aids in the absorption of your vitamins and minerals. Look at the liver like your body's internal filter, keeping the good and eliminating the bad. It detoxifies by metabolizing and/or secreting drugs, alcohol, and environmental toxins.

31) House Salad Juice

This is a great juice to drink on a day when you want to feel lean. Maybe you are going to the beach tomorrow and want to look good in that new bikini.

- 3 carrots
- ½ head lettuce
- ¼ red cabbage

Wash all of your veggies. Trim the tops off the carrots. Dice up the lettuce and cabbage to fit in your juicer.

32) Got Gray Hair?

This juice will you keep the gray away to come out another day!

- ¼ head lettuce
- ¼ head cabbage
- 2 carrots

Wash all your veggies. Trim the cabbage and the lettuce to fit inside the juicer.

33) Super Green Machine

This juice will get you cut up. When you are done drinking this juice, you will look like you dunked your abs in a bucket of knives. Not really, but you get my point.

- 1 cucumber
- 2 handfuls spinach
- 1 broccoli floret
- 2 kale leaves
- 1 lemon

Trim the skin off of your cucumber if it is not organic. Dice up the rest of your veggies so they fit in the juicer. Peel the skin off of the lemon if it is not organic.

34) Hair Rejuvenator

Worried about losing your hair? Ever notice how alfalfa sprouts look surprisingly like hair follicles? There are all types of people out there promising to regrow your hair, so why not try this organic, chemical-free one?

- 1 handful alfalfa sprouts
- 4 lettuce leaves
- 1 lemon
- 1 cucumber

Trim the tops off your carrots, and wash all the lettuce leaves and sprouts. Put the sprouts inside the lettuce leaf and juice.

35) Muscle Cramp Stopper

When cramping starts to happen, potassium can help aid you in muscle rejuvenation.

- 2 carrots
- 6 asparagus spears
- 6 celery stalks

Trim the tops off the carrots and wash your vegetables.

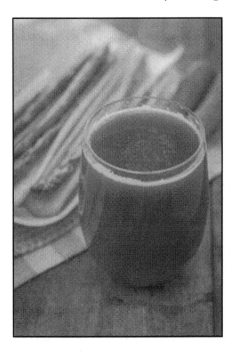

36) Infection Fighting and Virus Beater

Garlic is a natural antibiotic; it will help ward off any unwanted colds. Be careful not to add too much garlic, especially if you are going out on a hot date.

- 1 garlic clove
- 2 apples
- 2 carrots
- ½ beet
- 1 lemon

Skin the garlic and trim the tops off the carrots. Cut off the top of the beets and peel the lemon.

37) Jicama Juice

Are you afraid to admit that you don't know what jicama (pronounced "hik-a-muh") is? Well, fear not, I had no clue either. But it is very refreshing in juice!

- 1 slice jicama
- 3 carrots
- ½ beet
- 1 handful parsley

Jicama is great for an upset stomach. Make sure you wash all your vegetables and slice the tops off of your carrots.

38) Hopeful Heart

Great detoxifier juice and amazing for your heart and liver!

- 3 apples
- ½ beet

Wash all your vegetables. Peel the apple if it is not organic. Cut the top off of the beet and let the juicing begin.

39) L.A. Lung Juice

This is a great juice for detoxifying your lungs. If you are a little congested, this could free up some of the mucus that is clogging you up.

- 1 handful parsley
- 4 celery stalks
- 4 sprigs watercress

Wash your vegetables accordingly. Process them in the juicer.

Watercress—gram for gram—has a higher nutritional value then apples, broccoli, and tomatoes. The watercress has more C, B_1, B_6, K, E, iron, calcium, magnesium, manganese, and zinc. Only raw broccoli has more vitamin C and magnesium.

Watercress is bursting with beta-carotene and vitamin A—which, as well as being important antioxidants, are also needed for healthy skin and eyes—containing more than four times the amount of the other "power" foods. No wonder it is good for your lungs. Next time you are at the store, pick up some watercress.

40) Bone and Nail Health

The calcium content in these vegetables will strengthen your bones and nails.

- ½ cucumber
- 2 kale leaves
- ½ green bell pepper
- 1 lemon

Wash and trim your vegetables. Make sure you peel the lemon and cucumber if they are not organic.

41) Stamina Boost

The magnesium in this juice will provide long-lasting stamina. This juice adds intensity and extra "oomph!" to your workouts.

- ½ cucumber
- 2 bundles bok choy
- 4 carrots

Trim the tops off the carrots and peel your cucumber if it is not organic.

42) Pancrease Pump

Pump up the pancreas with this juice. The pancreas is in charge of insulin production. Insulin is responsible for breaking down glucose in your body. Pump up your insulin and burn body fat effectively and efficiently. What is good for the pancreas is good for the entire body.

- 2 apples
- 4 carrots
- 2 lettuce leaves
- 4 string beans
- 2 Brussels sprouts
- 1 handful sprouts

Make sure you wash all your vegetables. Put the sprouts inside the lettuce leaf and juice.

43) Go-Go Juice

This is a great juice to have in the morning before or after a workout. This is one of my favorite juices, getting me revved up and ready for the day. Simple to make but the rewards you get from the nutrients are incredible.

- ½ cucumber
- 1 lemon
- 1 ginger piece
- 2 apples
- 4 celery stalks

44) MEGA GREEN MAN (a.k.a. THE DAY SLAYER)

If you are in an energy slump, this is the juice for you, getting you revved up and ready to slay the day.

- 2 carrots
- 1 broccoli floret
- 2 collard green leaves
- 1-inch knob fresh ginger
- 2 handfuls spinach
- 1 handful dandelion greens
- ¼ beet
- 1 lemon

This juice is one of my personal favorites. Trim up the carrots so they fit in the juicer. If the lemon is not organic, trim the skin off that as well. Wash the rest of the vegetables with veggie wash and get ready to dominate life.

45) Hot Stuff

Jalapeno is great for opening up your circulatory system, ridding it from toxins.

- 1 jalapeno
- 1 cucumber
- ½ red bell pepper
- ½ beet

Wash your vegetables and peel the cucumber if it is not organic. Place the vegetables in the juicer.

46) Red Devil

Like spicy food? This juice is for you. Imagine your favorite Mexican dish in a glass. This one is great for headaches and congestion. I also love this one due to the fast-acting metabolism boost in the jalapeno and cayenne.

- 1 jalapeno
- 1 beet
- 2 red Swiss chard leaves
- 1 lemon
- 1 dash cayenne

Wash your vegetables. Cut the top off of the beet. Juice your vegetables and put a little cayenne pepper when stirring this juice up. (Stir up the juice with the pepper when done.)

Spicy foods can kick your metabolism into high gear. Juicing a tablespoon of chopped red or green chili pepper can temporarily boost your metabolic rate by 23 percent. This lasts for 30 to 45 minutes after eating.

Capsaicin (the chemical that puts the spice in your life and melts away body fat) also helps to inhibit inflammation and is beneficial in the treatment of arthritis and nerve disorders.

47) Hellatios Habanero

This one is at a level 10 on the hot gauge. If you like a burning sensation in your mouth, then this one is it. Habanero peppers contain amino acids that help regulate body functions. They contain vitamins A and C.

- 1 lemon
- 1 habanero pepper
- ½ cucumber
- 4 carrots
- 1 handful parsley

Granted, it's a little spicy, but it's an amazing juice to clean out your liver. Peel the lemon and trim the tops off of the carrots. Enjoy.

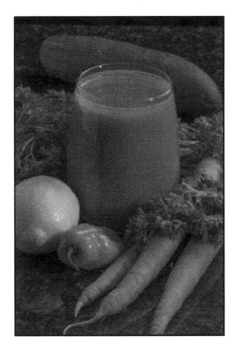

48) Sexy Skin Sap

This juice is great for colds and nausea. It is also great for smoother, age-defying skin.

- 1 lemon
- ½ cucumber
- 1 bunch watercress
- 2 carrots
- 1 ginger root

Wash all your vegetables and peel the cucumber and lemon if they are not organic.

49) Skin Revival

Are you ready to help diminish those fine lines and wrinkles? Have you been spending countless dollars on high-end beauty products and facials? Well, get ready to feast your face on this.

- 2 chard leaves
- 1 lemon
- 2 carrots
- ½ green bell pepper
- 2 kale leaves

Wash your vegetables. Cut the tops off of the carrots and peel the lemon if it is not organic. Process in the juicer.

50) Beet the Street Juice

This is a juice I like to drink before a long run. It gives me sustainable energy and it tastes delicious. Be careful at first, though, if you are not used to beets. Don't worry if your urine or bowel movements have a tinge of red/purple after consuming beets. They're just that powerful!

- 1 beet
- 4 celery stalks
- 1 lemon

Cut the tops off of the lemon and beet. Peel the lemon if it is not organic and process your vegetables in the juicer.

51) Zip Zap Zing Juice

This a powerful juice to drink before a meeting and when you need extra brainpower. This will give your brain the zip-zing that it needs to focus on the task at hand and get stuff done.

- ½ cucumber
- ½ beet
- 2 celery stalks
- ½ lemon
- 1 ginger root
- 1 handful cilantro
- 1 handful chard

Wash your vegetables. Place the herbs in the juicer halfway through to get the maximum benefit of the nutrients. Peel the lemon and cucumber if they are not organic. Cut the tops off of the cucumber and the beet. Process in the juicer.

52) Nite Nite Sleep Tight Juice

Having trouble sleeping? This will have you falling to sleep faster than you can count five sheep.

- 2 bundles bok choy
- 1 cucumber
- 2 handfuls spinach
- 1 lemon

Wash your vegetables. Peel the cucumber and lemon if they are not organic. Put the rest of the vegetables in the juicer and say good night.

53) The Situation Six-Pack

Get ready to pop out that sexy six-pack when chugging this alkaline goody.

- 2 carrots
- 1 cucumber
- ½ beet, with greens
- 3 handfuls spinach
- ½ lemon

Cut the tops off the carrots and peel the cucumber and lemon if they are not organic.

54) Extreme Juice

This juice is extreme! Coming out of the gates, we have the jalapeno that will open up your circulatory system and get you ready for the day—or anything else!

- 1 jalapeno pepper, seeded for less spice
- 1 cucumber
- 2 handfuls spinach
- 1 lemon
- 3 mustard green leaves

Make sure to peel the lemon and cucumber if they are not organic. This should make an 8-ounce glass of juice.

One natural ingredient in green juice recipes is chlorophyll, which is the product of plants turning light into energy for insects and animals to eat. Without chlorophyll, life as we know it would not exist. It has powerful detoxifying principles. It's great for the liver, which is necessary in purifying your body. Chlorophyll can also improve our blood quality due to its molecular makeup, similar to hemoglobin. It helps increase red blood cell count and increases the movement of oxygen throughout our blood. It also helps the repair and growth of all tissues in the body.

Parting Thoughts: You Make the Difference

> *"It was your character that got you out of bed, commitment that moved you into action, and ongoing discipline that enabled you to follow through and reach your destiny."*
>
> —Drew Canole

When I first started my exercise transformation, my body fat was a solid 17 percent. My exercise transformation started with going to the gym twice daily, where I pushed my body to the limits and maintained a healthy diet. It all resulted in trimming my stomach to a lean 12 percent in ninety days. However, when I started juicing daily, my gains increased substantially, continually lowering my body fat while building lean muscle.

Once the juice transformed my body's reception of nutrients, it enabled me to press out the water and toxins that were holding me back from my ultimate goal. This eventually allowed me to realize my potential sustainability of a body fat at or below 7 percent.

Maybe having a low body fat percentage is not your ideal goal, but optimum health is. If this is the case, the juice will help. However, exercise is a must! Even if it's just walking at first, you must take action. The hardest part for most people in the beginning of a regimen is to build up sustainability in doing so. The following six actions have helped me tremendously with my discipline and in my ability to take action. My hope is that they help you too!

1. Stop Being a Victim

Everyone who has a problem with their weight, overall physical health, or physique more often than not blames it on something outside of themselves: "I'm this way because of *this*."

Do you often find yourself saying or thinking these insignificant thoughts?

It's a hard pill to swallow when you realize *you're* the creator of everything that comes into your experience. Once you take ownership of it, you will begin to free yourself from all of the restrictions you've come up with in the past.

By not taking ownership, you end up rationalizing everything by telling yourself it isn't your fault and there isn't anything you can do about it, which ends up stunting your potential. For example, those extra three cookies you had Sunday after dinner. You might rationalize this indulgence by saying, "It's okay, I'll just do more cardio in the morning." The morning comes and the cardio never happens; sleep was too important, you have an extra-long day at work, etc.

You must take ownership and responsibility of the time you have in the present moment. Stop procrastinating. Once you master this discipline, you can get outside of your physical body and move this discipline to higher realms. Until then, you will be stuck on the island of blame with no escape.

Don't let yourself be a victim. Far too many people have the victim mentality. Don't try to rationalize why you are where you are right now by blaming other people and ill circumstances. Admit to yourself that you are in the situation you are in because of what YOU'VE done and no one else. Take control of your life. You can't go back to the past, but today you can start to create a new, healthy, enduring, and meaningful life.

2. Put Your Workouts on Automation

Wouldn't it be great to have your avatar venture into the gym every morning for you? For me personally, I have a morning routine that I follow. Perhaps this will encourage you to do the same.

- **5:30.** Wake up! (Ten minutes of gratitude. Drink one liter of water and grapefruit juice, equal parts. All of my gym clothes are laid out, ready to go. The easier I make it, the less I will fail.)
- **6:00:** Gym time. I have a timer set to give me one hour in the gym.
- **7:00–7:15:** Back home; juice time with a giant green drink.
- **7:30:** Meditate and read for one hour.
- **8:30:** Netti Pot, steam, and shower.
- **9:00:** Time to play. This is when I get to go to work.

The point of the automated morning routine is to form a lifelong habit of doing this. I call it a *success ritual*. When I miss a day or when I'm traveling, I miss my ritual because it sets me up for success every day. It wasn't always this way, I must admit. There was a time in my life when I DID NOT look forward to going to the gym, or even getting out of bed for that matter.

3. Set a Goal

If you really want to take your game to the next level, create urgency in your situation. Set a goal to run a race or some other type of competition. Far too often, we have no goals or plans, and we fail. Winston Churchill said it best: "By failing to prepare, you are preparing to fail." Create a plan and stick with it. Write out what you would like to accomplish—even if it is walking to the mailbox in two weeks, write it out.

4. Change Your Environment

It has been said that if you hang out with wolves you will become one. Or if you lie with dogs, you will get fleas. In any type of new regimen, some of the people in your life could subconsciously be holding you back. Understand that this behavior is not them; it is their own ego that is doing this. I'll make a bold claim: I can tell a person's fitness level by seeing five of the people they hang out with in their lives the most.

Who Are You Spending Your Time With?

Every cell in your body craves homeostasis, or balance. When you start to do something that is outside of the norm, some of the people in your life may not approve. Let's face it, not many of my friends crave broccoli and carrot juice at 6 a.m. before a workout on a Saturday morning.

What Do You Do When Faced with This Situation?

This is the best part—you make new friends. You don't have to get rid of your current friends; you just supplement them with these new individuals. In doing so, make sure they are the type of people who love broccoli and carrot juice, or at least accept you for you.

5. Turn It into a Game (advanced tactic)

One of my favorite things to do is to turn my routine into a game. I have a Gym Boss interval timer that I use to monitor my time. This puts me in a mode of "watching the stop clock." It's similar to the way a basketball player watches the clock at the end of each quarter and through the game, increasing his chances to win. The timer sits next to my bed and as soon as my gratitude moment is over, I jump out of bed excited and ready to take on the day.

Throughout my time getting ready, I'm cognizant of how much time I have to get to the gym, juice, have my gratitude moment, etc. This makes it fun each morning attempting to get more in and smash my time. The timer also causes me to focus 100 percent on what I'm doing right then and there. Many people multitask. When we multitask our brain function decreases by 45 percent. This is a surefire way to keep you engaged in one single activity, ensuring your success.

6. Intrinsic Value System

Once the habit is formed, it becomes part of your overall lifestyle and, in turn, your habits transcend into your values. If you can set your standards up to this level then you've got it. Having sustainability once you cherish and value this new routine should make it next to impossible for you to fail.

There will be times when you just can't make it to the gym, or go for a walk, run, jog, do yoga, etc. DO NOT beat yourself up for it. Always honor yourself for your courageous discipline and enjoy the day off. The great news is, once you master your physical body, you can use this same process in all other facets of your life: spiritual, financial, relational, communication, and so forth.

Conclusion

We can sit here and debate calories vs. carbs, or circuit training vs. long, slow running all day. But decidedly, if you don't have the mindset of the person you want to be, then you will never change. Real long-term change comes from within. Change your mind, change your body, and change your life.

Your Next Step

I Live to Give . . .

And the way I know I've delivered value to you is through your honest Amazon Review.

Please take three seconds and leave an Amazon review:
http://amzn.to/1FprrG0

Join Us!

Drew's Very Own Organic Superfood Greens Powder is NOW AVAILABLE!

http://bit.ly/1g1E3w6

Clean Up Your Gut And Improve Your Health...

bioticbalance.com

Join The Movement!

fitlifecertified.com

Need A Coach For Support and Accountability On Your Journey? We've Got You Covered!

fitlifevip.com/transformationcoaching

The FitLife Movement

We are in the business of changing lives. We are here to discover the way to vibrant health, strength, power, energy, and the very core of who we are as human beings. With new awareness and understanding often comes a desire to make a difference in the life of someone else. This is the foundation of the FitLife movement and something all of us are adamant about. We don't put out a book, an article, or anything if we don't believe 100 percent that it can impact someone's world for good.

If you're anything like us, you've got crazy goals, dreams, aspirations, and, at the very least, a hope that one day you will be truly happy and living the life of your dreams. Some of you are already there. Our goal is to help you all get there so we can continue moving forward together. This isn't just about me or your neighbor or your significant other or even you. It is about all of us. We're in this together, remember?

We know you have a desire to improve your life or you wouldn't be reading this book. We want you to know that we have absolute faith that you can reach your goals. We have already watched thousands of people transform their lives. The kind of transformation we are talking about is not only physical; but a mental, spiritual, truly life-changing transformation that connects people to their higher selves and to the Universe. This transformation is contagious and also very personal. Now it is your turn.

If your life has improved because of the material in this book, we would ask you to please help us share it with others who may also benefit from its content.

We are always looking for like-minded, heart-centered people around the globe to join our movement. If you're interested in this incredible opportunity to make a difference, contact our team and we'll be in touch! If you're interested in becoming a Certified FitLife Coach, we'd love to hear from you!

About the Author

Drew Canole is a rockstar in the world of fitness, nutrition and mindset, with a huge heart for others and doing his part to transform the world, one person at a time.

As the founder and CEO of FitLife.TV, he is committed to sharing educational, inspirational and entertaining videos and articles about health, fitness, healing and longevity.

Fueled by small town values with a big vision for a better planet, Drew aims to inspire and motivate others to search deep within themselves to create prosperous, healthy and enriching lifestyles. He truly believes that when you improve one life, you improve the world.

Drew and his team are committed to raising the vibration of the world we live in and leading the way for those ready and excited about improving their life and their health.

We're in this together.

Made in the USA
San Bernardino, CA
07 January 2016